# COMPLETE FITNESS

# The 9 Fundamentals of Fitness That Will Change Your Life

## Martin J Higgins

Table Of Contents

# What You'll Discover/Acquire from This Book

Complete fitness: The 9 Fundamentals of Fitness That Will Change Your Life  can offer a variety of benefits, including:

- Comprehensive Knowledge: This book cover various aspects of fitness, including exercise routines, nutrition, and mental well-being, providing a well-rounded understanding.

- Structured Workouts: You can learn effective workout routines tailored to different fitness goals, helping you achieve results more efficiently.

- Nutritional Guidance: This book offer insights into proper nutrition, helping you make healthier dietary choices to support your fitness journey.

- Motivation and Mindset: This book addresses the psychological aspects of fitness, offering tips to stay motivated, set goals, and develop a positive mindset.

- Injury Prevention: It will provide guidance on proper form and techniques, reducing the risk of injuries during workouts.

- Lifestyle Changes: This book often encourage healthier lifestyle changes beyond just exercise, fostering long-term well-being.

- Variety and Innovation: This book can introduce you to new exercises and training methods, keeping your workouts interesting and challenging.

# Introduction

Complete Fitness: The 9 Fundamentals of Fitness That Will Change Your Life is a comprehensive approach to achieving overall well-being through a balanced combination of physical exercise, healthy nutrition, and mental wellness. It emphasizes the integration of cardiovascular workouts, strength training, flexibility exercises, and mindfulness practices to improve physical fitness, mental clarity, and emotional resilience. By addressing various aspects of health, Complete Fitness aims to help individuals lead a more active, vibrant, and fulfilling life.

Complete fitness after the age of 40 is a crucial aspect of maintaining a healthy and active lifestyle as you age. As individuals reach this milestone, their bodies naturally undergo various changes, including a gradual decline in muscle mass, bone density, and metabolism. However, embracing a comprehensive approach to fitness can help counteract these effects and promote overall well-being. Complete fitness encompasses various components, including cardiovascular endurance, strength, flexibility, and balance. Here's an introduction to achieving and maintaining Complete fitness after the age of 40:

- Cardiovascular Fitness: Engaging in regular cardiovascular exercise, such as brisk walking, jogging, cycling, swimming, or dancing, helps improve heart health, lung capacity, and overall endurance. Aim for at least 150 minutes of moderate-intensity aerobic activity or 75 minutes of vigorous-intensity aerobic activity each week, spread over several days.

- Strength Training: As muscle mass naturally decreases with age, it's essential to include strength training or resistance exercises in your fitness routine. Weight lifting, bodyweight exercises, and resistance bands are effective ways to build and maintain muscle strength. Aim to target major muscle groups at least two days a week.

- Flexibility and Mobility: Maintaining good flexibility and mobility is vital for preventing injuries and maintaining a high quality of life. Incorporate stretching exercises or activities like yoga to enhance flexibility and keep your joints supple.

- Balance and Stability: Balance exercises become increasingly important with age to prevent falls and improve overall stability. Activities like Tai Chi, yoga, or even simply practicing standing on one leg can help enhance balance and coordination.

- Nutrition: Proper nutrition plays a significant role in total fitness. Focus on a well-balanced diet that includes a variety of nutrient-dense foods such as fruits, vegetables, lean proteins, whole grains, and healthy fats. Adequate hydration is also essential for overall health.

- Rest and Recovery: Giving your body enough time to rest and recover is crucial, especially as you age. Ensure you're getting enough quality sleep to support muscle recovery and overall well-being.

- Regular Health Check-ups: Regular visits to your healthcare provider are essential for monitoring your overall health, identifying any potential issues, and adjusting your fitness plan accordingly.

- Stress Management: Chronic stress can negatively impact your health and fitness. Incorporate stress-reduction techniques such as meditation, deep breathing, or engaging in hobbies you enjoy.

- Setting Realistic Goals: Set achievable fitness goals that consider your current fitness level and any health concerns. Gradually progress to more challenging activities to avoid overexertion and injuries.

- Consistency: Consistency is key to maintaining total fitness. Create a workout routine that you enjoy and can realistically stick to. Even small, regular efforts can lead to significant improvements over time.

Remember that fitness after 40 is a personal journey, and it's important to listen to your body and make adjustments as needed. Consulting with a fitness professional or healthcare provider can help you design a safe and effective fitness plan tailored to your individual needs and goals.

Chapter 1

# AGING CHANGES EVERYTHING

Absolutely, as we age, both our physical and mental attributes tend to change. Our bodies go through various physiological changes, such as changes in skin texture, muscle mass, bone density, and metabolism. Additionally, cognitive functions, memory, and even perspectives on life may evolve over time. It's a natural part of the human experience.

Indeed, aging is a natural process that brings about various physical, emotional, and cognitive changes over time.

## Aging's Impact On Bodybuilding

Aging can affect bodybuilding in several ways. As you age, your metabolism may slow down, making it more challenging to maintain muscle mass and control body fat. Hormone levels, such as testosterone, may decrease, impacting muscle growth and recovery. Joints and connective tissues might become more susceptible to injury or strain. However, with proper training, nutrition, and recovery strategies, it's still possible to continue bodybuilding and make progress as you age. Adjustments to your routine and expectations may be necessary to accommodate these changes.

## What's Happening to My Body?

When you're at the gym, your body goes through several physiological changes. Your heart rate increases to deliver more oxygen to your muscles, helping them work efficiently. Blood vessels dilate to enhance blood flow. Muscles contract and generate force to perform exercises. Your body temperature rises as you exert effort. Additionally, your brain releases endorphins, which are natural mood enhancers, contributing to the "feel-good" sensation often associated with exercise. Over time, consistent gym sessions can lead to improved strength, endurance, and overall fitness.

While at the gym, your body goes through various physiological changes. Your heart rate and breathing increase to supply more oxygen to your muscles. This helps fuel your muscles as you engage in exercises. Your muscles contract and relax to perform the movements, and this can lead to micro-tears in the muscle fibers. Over time, these tears repair and grow, contributing to muscle development and strength gains. Additionally, your body releases endorphins, which are natural painkillers that can create a sense of euphoria and reduce discomfort during exercise.

When you're at the gym, your body undergoes several physiological changes. Your heart rate increases to supply more oxygen and nutrients to your muscles, helping them work efficiently. Your muscles contract and generate force to perform exercises, leading to microtears in muscle fibers. This is a normal part of the muscle-building process. Additionally, your body releases endorphins, which are feel-good chemicals that can reduce pain perception and boost your mood. Over time, consistent gym workouts can lead to increased muscle strength, endurance, and improved overall fitness.

## What Fitness Can Do For You

Fitness can offer numerous benefits, such as improved physical health, increased energy levels, better mood, stress reduction, and enhanced overall quality of life. Regular exercise can help maintain a healthy weight, boost cardiovascular health, strengthen muscles and bones, and promote better sleep. It also has the potential to enhance cognitive function and reduce the risk of chronic diseases.

Fitness can offer numerous benefits for both your physical and mental well-being:

1. Improved Physical Health: Regular exercise enhances cardiovascular health, strengthens muscles and bones, and improves flexibility. It can also help manage weight, lower the risk of chronic conditions like heart disease, diabetes, and obesity, and boost your immune system.

2. Increased Energy: Engaging in physical activity increases your overall energy levels by promoting better circulation and oxygen flow throughout the body.

3. Better Mental Health: Exercise triggers the release of endorphins, which are natural mood lifters. It can reduce symptoms of anxiety and depression, improve cognitive function, and enhance overall mental clarity.

4. Stress Reduction: Physical activity can act as a stress reliever. It helps reduce the levels of stress hormones in your body and can contribute to better emotional resilience.

5. Enhanced Sleep: Regular exercise can lead to better sleep quality and help combat insomnia. However, it's recommended not to exercise too close to bedtime.

6. Increased Confidence: Achieving fitness goals can boost self-esteem and body image, leading to increased self-confidence in various aspects of life.

7. Social Interaction: Participating in group fitness activities or sports can provide opportunities for social interaction, fostering a sense of community and belonging.

8. Cognitive Benefits: Exercise has been shown to improve cognitive function, memory, and concentration. It can also help reduce the risk of cognitive decline and certain neurodegenerative diseases.

9. Longevity: Leading an active lifestyle is associated with a longer lifespan and improved overall quality of life as you age.

10. Preventive Measures: Regular exercise can play a role in preventing various health issues, such as osteoporosis, certain types of cancer, and metabolic disorders.

11. Weight Management: Combining exercise with a balanced diet can aid in weight loss or weight maintenance by increasing calorie expenditure and muscle mass.

12. Improved Posture and Balance: Engaging in exercises that focus on core strength, flexibility, and balance can lead to better posture and reduced risk of falls, especially as you age.

13. Heart Health: Cardiovascular exercises like running, swimming, and cycling improve heart health by increasing heart rate and improving circulation.

14. Better Immune Function: Regular moderate exercise can enhance immune function and reduce the risk of infections.

15. Enhanced Creativity: Physical activity has been linked to increased creativity and problem-solving abilities, likely due to its positive effects on brain function.

16. Pain Management: Exercise can alleviate certain types of chronic pain, such as back pain and arthritis, by promoting muscle strength and flexibility.

It's important to note that the benefits of fitness are best achieved through consistent, balanced, and personalized routines that suit your individual needs and preferences. Always consult with a healthcare professional before starting a new fitness regimen, especially if you have any underlying health conditions.

## The 9 Foundations of Complete Fitness

The "Nine Foundations of Complete Fitness" is a concept popularized by the American Council on Exercise (ACE) to provide a comprehensive approach to achieving overall fitness. These foundations encompass various aspects of physical well-being. Here they are:

1. **Aerobic Endurance**: This refers to the ability of your cardiovascular system to transport oxygen efficiently during sustained physical activity, improving heart and lung health.

2. **Muscular Strength**: It involves the maximum force a muscle or muscle group can generate, contributing to better overall body strength and functionality.

3. **Muscular Endurance**: This foundation focuses on the capacity of muscles to perform repeated contractions over time, enhancing activities that require sustained effort.

4. **Flexibility**: Flexibility helps maintain a full range of motion in your joints and muscles, reducing the risk of injury and improving overall movement quality.

5. **Mobility**: Mobility goes beyond flexibility, encompassing the ability to move joints through their full range of motion actively, ensuring functional movement patterns.

6. **Body Composition**: This involves the proportion of lean body mass (muscles, bones, organs) to body fat, indicating overall health and fitness.

7. **Balance**: Balance training enhances stability and coordination, which is vital for preventing falls and maintaining efficient movement.

8. **Core Stability**: A strong core supports your spine and pelvis, aiding in overall posture, stability, and injury prevention.

9. **Reaction Time and Speed**: These foundations focus on the ability to react quickly and move swiftly, improving coordination and athletic performance.

By incorporating exercises and activities that address each of these foundations, you can work towards a well-rounded fitness routine that promotes holistic health and well-being.

# Chapter 2
## DEVELOPING A MINDSET FOR SUCCESS

Developing a mindset for success involves cultivating positive beliefs, setting clear goals, staying persistent, embracing challenges as opportunities to learn, and maintaining a growth-oriented attitude. It's also essential to practice self-discipline, manage time effectively, and surround yourself with supportive people and resources. Remember, success is a journey that requires continuous learning and adaptation.

### Visualizing Power

Visualization is a powerful technique where you create mental images of your goals, desires, or scenarios you want to manifest. It can help enhance focus, motivation, and overall performance by training your mind to believe in your capabilities and objectives. Many successful individuals use visualization as a tool to achieve their aspirations.

Visualization is a potent mental tool that involves creating vivid mental images to achieve goals, enhance performance, or manage stress. By picturing desired outcomes, individuals can stimulate motivation, improve focus, and increase self-confidence. This technique taps into the brain's ability to blur the line between imagination and reality, thereby influencing behavior and positively impacting various aspects of life, such as sports, education, and personal development.

Visualization is a powerful technique that involves creating detailed mental images of desired outcomes or goals. It taps into the brain's ability to simulate experiences, enhancing motivation, focus, and performance. By vividly imagining success, individuals can increase their confidence, reduce anxiety, and improve their chances of achieving their objectives. This technique is commonly used in sports, personal development, and even medical practices to harness the mind's capacity to shape reality through the power of positive imagery.

# Smart Goal Setting Guide

SMART goal setting is a framework used to create clear and achievable goals. SMART stands for Specific, Measurable, Achievable, Relevant, and Time-bound. It's a way to ensure that goals are well-defined, trackable, realistic, and have a clear timeframe for completion. By following the SMART criteria, individuals and businesses can increase their chances of success and effective progress tracking.

SMART goal setting is an effective approach for achieving total fitness:

- **Specific**: Define a clear goal, such as losing a certain amount of weight, improving cardiovascular endurance, or increasing muscle strength.

- **Measurable**: Set quantifiable parameters to track progress, like tracking body measurements, monitoring heart rate during workouts, or recording the number of push-ups you can do.

- **Achievable**: Ensure that your goal is realistic and attainable given your age, fitness level, and any potential health concerns. Consult a doctor or fitness professional if needed.

- **Relevant**: Choose goals that align with your overall health and well-being, considering the specific needs and challenges that come with being over 40.

- **Time-Bound**: Set a specific timeframe for achieving your goal. For instance, aim to lose a certain amount of weight within six months or complete a 5k run in three months.

Remember, gradual progress and consistency are key. It's essential to incorporate a balanced mix of cardiovascular exercises, strength training, flexibility work, and proper nutrition into your routine. Also, consider seeking guidance from a fitness professional to create a personalized plan tailored to your age and fitness level.

## Embrace Exercise Gradually

Embracing exercise can be a gradual process. Start by finding activities that genuinely interest you and align with your preferences. Set achievable goals, track your progress, and celebrate your accomplishments along the way. Consistency is key, and over time, the positive effects of exercise on your mood, energy levels, and overall well-being can help foster a genuine appreciation for physical activity.

Embracing exercise gradually is a sensible approach to avoid injury and ensure long-term commitment. Here's a list of steps to help you get started:

1. **Assess Your Current Fitness Level:** Understand your current physical condition and any limitations you might have. This will help you choose the right type and intensity of exercise.

2. **Set Realistic Goals**: Establish achievable short-term and long-term goals. These could be related to weight loss, strength gain, flexibility improvement, or overall fitness enhancement.

3. **Choose Activities You Enjoy:** Opt for exercises that you find enjoyable and interesting. This increases the likelihood of sticking with them over the long run.

4. **Start Slowly**: Begin with low-intensity workouts to give your body time to adjust. This might include brisk walks, gentle yoga, or light cardio.

5. **Warm Up and Cool Down**: Always warm up with dynamic stretches before exercising and cool down with static stretches afterward. This helps prevent muscle strains and soreness.

6. **Gradually Increase Intensity**: Slowly increase the intensity, duration, or frequency of your workouts. Aim for around 10% increments every week to avoid overexertion.

7. **Mix Up Workouts:** Incorporate variety into your routine to prevent boredom and overuse injuries. Combine cardiovascular, strength, and flexibility exercises.

8. **Listen to Your Body**: Pay attention to how your body responds to exercise. If you feel pain, discomfort, or excessive fatigue, it's a sign to dial back or take a break.

9. **Rest and Recovery**: Allow your body sufficient time to recover between workouts. Rest days are essential to prevent burnout and overtraining.

10. **Stay Hydrated and Eat Well:** Proper nutrition and hydration are crucial to support your exercise efforts. Consume a balanced diet and drink enough water.

11. **Monitor Progress**: Keep track of your workouts, noting improvements in strength, endurance, and overall well-being. This can be motivating and help you stay committed.

12. **Consult Professionals**: If you have pre-existing health conditions or concerns, consult a doctor or fitness professional before starting a new exercise regimen.

Note; the key is consistency. Gradually embracing exercise ensures a sustainable approach that leads to long-term benefits for your health and well-being.

## Exercise Habit Building Guides

Exercise habit building is a process that involves consistently engaging in physical activity to improve your overall fitness and well-being. Here are the steps to help you understand and establish this habit:

1. ***Start Small***: Begin with manageable exercise sessions that fit into your daily routine. This could be as simple as a 10-minute walk or a quick set of push-ups.

2. ***Set Clear Goals***: Define specific and achievable goals for your exercise routine. Whether it's improving cardiovascular health, building muscle, or losing weight, having clear objectives can keep you motivated.

3. ***Choose Enjoyable Activities:*** Engage in activities you enjoy to increase the likelihood of sticking with them. It could be jogging, dancing, swimming, or playing a sport.

4. ***Create a Schedule***: Establish a consistent exercise schedule that aligns with your daily routine. This makes it easier to form a habit and reduces the chances of skipping workouts.

5. ***Accountability:*** Consider exercising with a friend, joining a fitness class, or using fitness apps to help you stay accountable and motivated.

6. ***Gradual Progression***: As your fitness level improves, gradually increase the intensity and duration of your workouts to avoid burnout or injuries.

7. ***Track Your Progress***: Keep track of your workouts and progress. This helps you see how far you've come and provides a sense of accomplishment.

8. ***Reward Yourself***: Celebrate your achievements and milestones to reinforce positive behavior and make the habit more enjoyable.

9. ***Overcome Barriers***: Identify and address obstacles that might hinder your exercise routine. Lack of time, fatigue, or external factors can be overcome with proper planning.

10.      ***Rest and Recovery***: Give your body enough time to rest and recover. Overtraining can lead to burnout and injury, so listen to your body's signals.

11. ***Mindset Shift***: View exercise as an essential part of your lifestyle rather than a chore. Cultivate a positive attitude toward physical activity.

12. ***Adaptability***: Be flexible with your routine. Life can get busy, so having the ability to adapt your workout plan when needed will help you stay consistent.

13. ***Long-Term Focus***: Building the exercise habit is a long-term commitment. Embrace the journey and recognize that results may take time to show.

Remember that building a habit takes time and effort, but the benefits to your physical and mental health are well worth it. Stay patient, stay consistent, and enjoy the process of becoming a healthier version of yourself.

## Energy Systems For Fitness

Fitness energy systems refer to the various physiological processes that provide the energy needed for physical activities. The three primary energy systems are the phosphagen system, glycolytic system, and aerobic system. The phosphagen system provides quick bursts of energy for short, high-intensity activities, the glycolytic system provides energy for medium-intensity activities, and the aerobic system supplies energy for prolonged, lower-intensity activities. Different types of exercises rely on these energy systems to varying degrees.

There are three primary energy systems that your body uses during physical activity: the phosphagen system, the glycolytic system, and the aerobic sysystem.

1. **Phosphagen System (ATP-PCr System):** This system provides immediate energy for short bursts of intense activity, such as weightlifting or sprinting. It uses stored creatine phosphate and ATP (adenosine triphosphate) in muscles to generate energy quickly. However, this system is limited and can only sustain activity for about 10-15 seconds.

2. **Glycolytic System (Anaerobic System):** When activity continues beyond the duration supported by the phosphagen system, the glycolytic system takes over. It breaks down glucose (or stored glycogen) into ATP through a process called glycolysis. This system provides energy for activities like high-intensity intervals or medium-duration efforts. It doesn't require oxygen but produces lactic acid as a byproduct, leading to muscle fatigue.

3. **Aerobic System (Oxidative System):** For longer-lasting activities like jogging, cycling, or endurance events, the aerobic system is the primary source of energy. It relies on oxygen to break down carbohydrates, fats, and, to a lesser extent, proteins, yielding ATP through a process called cellular respiration. This system is more efficient and sustainable compared to the other two but takes longer to produce energy.

Each system contributes to different types of physical activities, and they work together depending on the intensity and duration of the exercise. It's important to train all these systems to improve overall fitness and performance.

# The Importance of Your Fitness Training

Fitness training is crucial for overall health and well-being. It helps improve cardiovascular health, build muscle strength, enhance flexibility, and boost endurance. Regular exercise also contributes to weight management, reduces the risk of chronic diseases like diabetes and heart disease, and promotes mental well-being by releasing endorphins. Additionally, fitness training can improve posture, bone density, and balance, reducing the risk of injuries as you age. It's an essential part of maintaining a healthy lifestyle.

Here are six important benefits of fitness training:

1. ***Improved Physical Health***: Fitness training helps enhance cardiovascular health, strengthen muscles, and improve flexibility. It can lower the risk of chronic conditions like heart disease, diabetes, and obesity.

2. ***Weight Management:*** Regular exercise helps burn calories, aiding in weight loss or maintenance. Combined with a balanced diet, fitness training contributes to achieving and maintaining a healthy weight.

3. ***Increased Energy Levels***: Engaging in regular physical activity boosts energy levels by improving blood circulation and oxygen delivery to cells. This results in increased stamina and reduced feelings of fatigue.

4. ***Mental Well-being***: Exercise releases endorphins, which are natural mood enhancers. Fitness training has been linked to reduced stress, anxiety, and depression, promoting overall mental well-being.

5. ***Enhanced Cognitive Function:*** Physical activity supports brain health by improving blood flow to the brain, promoting the growth of new neurons, and enhancing cognitive functions like memory, concentration, and problem-solving.

6. ***Social Interaction and Confidence***: Participating in group fitness classes or sports activities provides opportunities for social interaction, fostering a sense of community and belonging. Regular exercise also boosts self-esteem and confidence through accomplishments and improved body image.

Remember, individual results may vary, and it's important to tailor your fitness routine to your personal needs and goals.

## Heart Rate

Heart rate is a crucial metric in fitness as it reflects the intensity of your workout. It's typically measured in beats per minute (BPM). Different heart rate zones correspond to various exercise intensities, such as fat burning, aerobic training, and anaerobic training. Monitoring your heart rate during exercise can help you optimize your workouts and track your progress.

Imagine your heart as the engine that powers your body during a workout. Your heart rate, which is the number of times your heart beats per minute, is like the rhythm of that engine. When you start exercising, your body demands more oxygen and energy. In response, your heart beats faster to pump oxygen-rich blood to your muscles, kind of like a fuel delivery system.

As you push harder, your heart rate increases even more, just like how a car's engine revs up when you accelerate. This increased heart rate helps deliver nutrients to your muscles and removes waste products. It's a bit like the engine running at full throttle to keep up with the demands of your workout.

Monitoring your heart rate during fitness training is like watching the dashboard of your car. It gives you valuable information about the intensity of your exercise. Are you cruising along at a steady pace or sprinting at full speed? By paying attention to your heart rate, you can adjust your workout to stay in the optimal zone for your goals. Whether it's improving endurance, burning fat, or building strength, your heart rate is the indicator that guides your fitness journey.

# Chapter 3
## STRENGTH -YOU ARE STRONGER THAN YOU KNOW

Amid life's trials and challenges, you stand as a beacon of resilience, a testament to the hidden wellspring of strength within you. It's in those moments when doubt and weariness try to take hold that your true power emerges, unwavering and unyielding. Like a mighty oak weathering storms, your inner strength runs deep, drawing from the experiences, lessons, and triumphs that have shaped you.

Within the tapestry of your journey, threads of determination and courage are woven, creating a mosaic of endurance that paints a picture of unwavering tenacity. Your strength is not solely defined by physical might, but by the fortitude that allows you to push through mental barriers and rise above emotional tides.

Every step forward, no matter how small, is a testament to your innate strength. The battles you've faced and conquered are the testament of your ability to overcome, to adapt, and to thrive. Often, it's when faced with the unknown that your true strength comes into focus, as you navigate uncharted waters and emerge with newfound wisdom and confidence.

So remember, you are stronger than you know. Your strength is a tapestry of past triumphs, present determination, and future potential. Embrace it, channel it, and let it guide you through the chapters of your life, reminding you that you have the power to conquer obstacles and flourish in the face of adversity.

## Strength Training Pyramids

Strength training pyramids are a workout technique where you gradually increase and then decrease the weight lifted during a workout session. This approach helps to target muscle fatigue while allowing for recovery during the workout. Typically, the pyramid consists of sets with ascending and descending repetitions or weights. For example, you might start with a light weight for higher reps, increase the weight while decreasing reps, and then reverse the process. This method can help challenge muscles and promote muscle growth.

Strength training pyramids are a method often used in weightlifting and resistance training to structure the progression of weights and repetitions during a workout. There are different types of strength training pyramids, including ascending, descending, and triangle/pyramid.

**Ascending Pyramid:**
In an ascending pyramid, you start with a lighter weight and gradually increase the weight with each set while decreasing the number of repetitions. For example:

- *Set 1:* 12 reps x 50kg
- *Set 2:* 10 reps x 60kg
- *Set 3:* 8 reps x 70kg

**Descending Pyramid:**
In a descending pyramid, you start with a heavier weight and decrease the weight with each set while increasing the number of repetitions. For example:

- *Set 1*: 8 reps x 80kg
- *Set 2:* 10 reps x 70kg
- *Set 3*: 12 reps x 60kg

**Triangle/Pyramid Pyramid**:
In a triangle pyramid, you increase the weight for a few sets and then decrease it, creating a triangular pattern. For example:

- *Set 1:* 8 reps x 70kg
- *Set 2:* 6 reps x 80kg
- *Set 3:* 4 reps x 90kg
- *Set 4:* 6 reps x 80kg

- ***Set 5:*** 8 reps x 70kg

These pyramids help provide variation in intensity during a workout, which can be beneficial for muscle adaptation and growth. They can also be adjusted based on individual goals, such as strength, hypertrophy, or endurance. Always ensure proper form and technique while performing these exercises to avoid injury.

## Movement Quality

Movement quality in fitness refers to the way exercises and movements are performed. It focuses on factors like proper form, alignment, stability, and control. Emphasizing movement quality helps prevent injuries, enhances muscle activation, and improves overall effectiveness of workouts.

Movement quality in body fitness refers to the manner in which you perform exercises and movements, focusing on technique, control, and alignment. It's not just about completing a movement, but doing it correctly and efficiently. Here are a few aspects of movement quality:

1. **Alignment**: Proper alignment ensures that your body is in the correct position during exercises, minimizing the risk of injury and maximizing muscle engagement. This involves maintaining a neutral spine, keeping joints stacked, and avoiding excessive deviations.

2. **Control**: Controlling the movement throughout its full range of motion helps prevent jerky or abrupt motions that can lead to strain. It also enhances muscle activation and improves overall muscle strength.

3. **Range of Motion**: Working through a full range of motion helps maintain joint health, flexibility, and mobility. However, it's important to avoid pushing into ranges that cause discomfort or compromise form.

4. **Breathing**: Proper breathing during exercise supports stability and energy delivery to muscles. It's often advised to exhale during the most exerting phase of a movement and inhale during the less intense phase.

5. **Stability and Balance:** Maintaining stability and balance during exercises challenges your core muscles and improves overall coordination. This is particularly important when performing unilateral (single-sided) exercises.

6. **Mind-Muscle Connection**: Focusing your attention on the muscle being worked enhances muscle activation and engagement. This connection can lead to better results and improved muscle recruitment.

7. **Posture**: Maintaining good posture during exercises and daily activities supports muscle balance, prevents strain, and promotes overall body alignment.

8. **Progressive Loading**: Gradually increasing the resistance or intensity of exercises helps build strength without compromising movement quality. Rushing through progressions can lead to poor technique and potential injury.

9. **Variation and Adaptation**: Incorporating a variety of movements prevents overuse injuries and promotes balanced muscle development. Your body adapts to movements, so introducing new ones challenges it in different ways.

10. **Recovery and Rest:** Allowing adequate time for recovery and rest is essential to prevent overtraining, which can negatively impact movement quality due to fatigue and reduced focus.

Focusing on movement quality not only reduces the risk of injury but also improves the effectiveness of your workouts. It's a foundation for building strength, flexibility, and overall fitness in a sustainable and safe manner.

## Exercise Selection

Absolutely, exercise selection is a crucial step in creating an effective workout routine. It's important to choose exercises that align with your fitness goals, target the muscle groups you want to work on, and suit your fitness level.

Exercise selection in fitness involves choosing specific exercises to include in a workout routine. It's crucial to tailor the exercises to your goals, fitness level, and any limitations you might have. Here are some key points to consider when selecting exercises:

1. **Goals**: Determine your fitness goals, such as building strength, increasing endurance, improving flexibility, or targeting specific muscle groups. Choose exercises that align with these objectives.

2. **Muscle Groups**: Include exercises that work various muscle groups to create a well-rounded routine. Compound exercises like squats, deadlifts, and bench presses engage multiple muscles at once.

3. **Progression**: Incorporate exercises that allow for progressive overload, which means gradually increasing the resistance or intensity over time. This stimulates muscle growth and strength gains.

4. **Variety**: Avoid monotony by including a mix of exercises to keep your routine engaging. This can also prevent plateaus and overuse injuries.

5. **Skill Level**: Choose exercises appropriate for your fitness level. Beginners might start with bodyweight movements and simpler

resistance exercises, while experienced individuals can include more complex lifts.

6. **Equipment**: Consider the equipment you have access to. Whether it's free weights, machines, resistance bands, or bodyweight exercises, make sure you can perform the chosen exercises safely and effectively.

7. **Functional Movements**: Select exercises that mimic real-life movements to improve overall functionality and coordination. These movements can enhance daily activities and sports performance.

8. **Rest and Recovery:** Allow sufficient time for recovery by not overloading certain muscle groups with too many exercises. Adequate rest is essential for muscle repair and growth.

9. **Flexibility and Mobility**: Incorporate exercises that improve flexibility and joint mobility. Yoga, dynamic stretches, and mobility drills can be beneficial.

10. **Injury Prevention:** Avoid exercises that exacerbate existing injuries or limitations. Consult a fitness professional or healthcare provider if you're unsure about exercise suitability.

11. **Time**: Consider the duration of your workout. Some exercises require more time and attention than others. Balance your routine based on the time you have available.

12. **Cardiovascular Conditioning:** Include cardiovascular exercises like running, cycling, or swimming to improve your heart health and endurance.

Remember, a well-balanced exercise selection should address your individual needs and preferences, taking into account your physical condition, goals, and the resources available to you. Consulting with a itness professional can help you create a tailored workout plan that aligns with your objectives.

## Fitness Concepts: Intensity, Volume & Frequency

In fitness, intensity, volume, and frequency are key concepts that help determine the effectiveness of a workout routine:

1. **Intensity**: This refers to how hard you're working during a workout. It's often measured as a percentage of your maximum effort. High intensity means pushing yourself close to your limits, which can lead to improvements in strength, endurance, and overall fitness. Low intensity is less demanding and is often used for recovery or light exercise.

2. **Volume**: Volume is the total amount of work you do during a workout. It's typically calculated by multiplying the number of sets, reps, and weight lifted. A higher volume can lead to muscle growth and increased strength, but it also requires adequate recovery time to avoid overtraining.

3. **Frequency**: Frequency is how often you engage in a specific type of exercise or workout. It's important to find a balance that allows for proper recovery between sessions. Too much frequency can lead to burnout or injuries, while too little might not provide enough stimulus for progress.

Finding the right balance between intensity, volume, and frequency is essential for achieving your fitness goals, whether you're aiming to build muscle, improve cardiovascular health, or enhance overall fitness. It's important to gradually progress and listen to your body to avoid overexertion and ensure sustainable results.

## Tracking Your Fitness Progression

To track your progression in total fitness, follow these steps:

1. Set Clear Goals: Define specific fitness goals, such as weight loss, muscle gain, or improved cardiovascular endurance.

2. Record Baseline Measurements: Take initial measurements of your weight, body measurements (waist, hips, etc.), and fitness levels (e.g., how many push-ups or sit-ups you can do, your running time for a certain distance).

3. Keep a Workout Journal: Maintain a record of your workouts, noting the exercises, sets, reps, and weights used. This will help you monitor your progress and make adjustments as needed.

4. Regular Assessments: Periodically reevaluate your fitness levels. This could involve repeating the initial measurements and fitness tests every few weeks or months.

5. Track Nutrition: Keep a food diary to monitor your dietary habits and ensure you're fueling your body properly to support your fitness goals.

6. Monitor Performance: Track your progress during workouts. For instance, if you're lifting weights, you might notice that you're lifting heavier weights or performing more repetitions over time.

7. Use Fitness Apps or Wearables: Utilize fitness apps or wearables that can track your workouts, steps, heart rate, and more. These tools can provide valuable data on your progress.

8. Listen to Your Body: Pay attention to how your body feels. Increased energy levels, improved sleep quality, and enhanced mood can all be indicators of fitness progress.

9. Adjust Your Plan: Modify your workout routine, nutrition, and goals as necessary based on your progress. Plateaus are common, so changing things up can help you continue advancing.

10. Celebrate Achievements: Recognize and celebrate your accomplishments along the way, whether it's hitting a new personal best or reaching a milestone in your fitness journey.

Remember that fitness progression takes time and consistency. By staying dedicated and tracking your efforts, you'll be able to see the positive changes you're making over time.

## Rest, Interval and Tempo

Rest, interval, and tempo are important concepts in total fitness training:

- **Rest**: Adequate rest is crucial to allow your body to recover and repair after workouts. It's during rest periods that your muscles grow stronger and your body replenishes its energy stores. Make sure to incorporate rest days into your routine to prevent overtraining and reduce the risk of injury.

- **Interval Training**: Interval training involves alternating between periods of high-intensity exercise and periods of lower-intensity or rest. This approach can be very effective for improving cardiovascular fitness, burning calories, and boosting metabolism. It's a versatile technique that can be used in various forms of exercise, such as running, cycling, or strength training.

- **Tempo Training**: Tempo training, also known as tempo runs or tempo workouts, focuses on running or exercising at a sustained, challenging pace that's faster than your regular pace but still manageable. This type of training helps improve your lactate threshold, which is the point at which lactic acid builds up in your muscles. By training at this threshold, you can increase your body's ability to tolerate and clear lactic acid, leading to improved endurance.

Remember, the balance between these concepts will depend on your fitness goals and the type of exercise you're doing. It's important to consult with a fitness professional to create a well-rounded and effective training plan that incorporates proper rest, interval, and tempo training.

## Strength Training Basics

Strength training involves a systematic approach to improve muscle strength and endurance. It typically includes resistance exercises like weightlifting, bodyweight exercises, and resistance bands. To implement it effectively, start with a warm-up, focus on compound exercises, gradually increase weights, maintain proper form, and allow sufficient rest between sessions. Always consult a fitness professional if you're new to strength training to ensure safety and effectiveness.

Here are some basic principles of strength training:

- **Progressive Overload**: This involves gradually increasing the resistance or weight you lift over time. It challenges your muscles and encourages growth and strength gains.

- **Compound Movements**: Focus on compound exercises like squats, deadlifts, bench presses, and overhead presses. These work multiple muscle groups simultaneously, leading to efficient overall strength development.

- **Isolation Exercises**: These target specific muscles and help in balanced development. Examples include bicep curls, tricep extensions, and calf raises.

- **Sets and Repetitions**: A typical strength training session involves performing a certain number of sets (groups of repetitions) for each exercise. A common setup is 3-4 sets of 8-12 repetitions per set.

- **Rest and Recovery:** Give your muscles time to recover between workouts. Usually, 48 hours is recommended before targeting the same muscle group again.

- **Proper Form**: Maintaining proper form is crucial to prevent injuries and maximize effectiveness. It's better to lift a lighter weight with good form than a heavier weight with poor form.

- **Warm-up and Cool-down**: Warming up prepares your muscles for the workout, while cooling down helps reduce post-workout soreness and stiffness.

- **Nutrition**: A balanced diet with adequate protein is essential for muscle growth and repair. Stay hydrated and consider post-workout nutrition.

- **Rest Days:** Schedule rest days to allow your body to recover and adapt. Rest is essential for avoiding burnout and overtraining.

- **Consistency**: Strength gains come with consistent training over time. It's better to have a consistent routine rather than sporadic intense sessions.

Remember to start with an appropriate weight that challenges you but allows you to maintain proper form. If you're new to strength training, consider consulting a fitness professional to create a tailored plan based on your goals and fitness level.

### Sample Workouts

Here are a couple of sample workouts for both cardio and strength training:

**Cardio Workout:**

*Interval Running*: Warm up with a 5-minute jog, then alternate between 1 minute of sprinting and 2 minutes of brisk walking for a total of 20 minutes. Cool down with a 5-minute walk.

*Cycling Intervals*: Warm up for 5 minutes, then alternate between 3 minutes of fast pedaling and 2 minutes of slower pedaling for a total of 25 minutes. Cool down with 5 minutes of easy cycling.

**Cardio and Fat Loss:**
- Jogging or Running: 20-30 minutes
- Jumping Jacks: 3 sets of 1 minute
- Burpees: 3 sets of 10 reps
- Cycling: 20-30 minutes
- High-Intensity Interval Training (HIIT): Alternate between 30 seconds of intense exercise and 30 seconds of rest for 10-15 minutes.

**Muscle Building:**

- Bench Press: 4 sets of 6-8 reps
- Pull-ups or Lat Pulldowns: 4 sets of 8-10 reps
- Deadlifts: 3 sets of 5 reps
- Leg Press: 3 sets of 8 reps
- Bicep Curls: 3 sets of 10-12 reps

**Strength Training Workout:**

*Full-Body Circuit*: Perform 3 rounds of the following exercises with minimal rest between them:

- Squats: 3 sets of 8-10 reps
- Push-ups: 3 sets of 10-12 reps
- Bent-over Rows: 3 sets of 8-10 reps

- Lunges: 3 sets of 10 reps each leg
- Plank: 3 sets of 20-30 seconds
- Squats (12 reps)
- Push-ups (10 reps)
- Bent-over Rows (12 reps)
- Lunges (10 reps each leg)
- Plank (hold for 30 seconds)

***Upper Body Focus***: Do 4 sets of the following exercises:

- Bench Press (8 reps)
- Pull-ups or Lat Pulldowns (10 reps)
- Dumbbell Shoulder Press (10 reps)
- Tricep Dips (12 reps)

Remember to warm up before starting any workout and cool down afterwards. Adjust the weights and intensity based on your fitness level, and it's always a good idea to consult a fitness professional before starting a new exercise routine.

## Warming up/Cooling down Essentials

Imagine you're about to embark on a fitness journey. Think of warming up as the gentle sunrise before a beautiful day and cooling down as the calming sunset after an active day.

**Warming up**: This is like slowly turning on the engine of a car before you hit the road. It's a short period of low-intensity activity that gets your heart rate gradually up, your muscles warmed, and your joints lubricated. Picture yourself doing some light jogging, arm swings, leg stretches, and body rotations. This prepares your body for the more intense exercise that's coming up, reducing the risk of injury and improving your performance.

**Cooling down:** After a vigorous workout, cooling down is like guiding your body back to a state of calm. It's a time to gently slow down your heart rate and let your body return to its resting state. Think of it as giving your muscles a chance to catch their breath. Imagine yourself doing slow stretches, deep breathing, and perhaps some gentle yoga poses. Cooling down helps prevent dizziness and muscle cramps, promotes flexibility, and aids in the recovery process.

So, just like a sunrise and a sunset frame your day, warming up and cooling down frame your fitness routine, ensuring you start and finish on a healthy note.

# Chapter 4
## FLEXIBLY-STRENGTH TO IMPRESS

Flexibility is an important component of total fitness. It involves the ability of your joints and muscles to move through a full range of motion. Incorporating stretching exercises, yoga, or Pilates into your fitness routine can help improve flexibility, enhance joint mobility, and reduce the risk of injuries. Remember to warm up before stretching and to practice proper techniques to avoid overstretching or causing harm.

## What is Flexibility?
Flexibility: This refers to the ability of your muscles and joints to move through their full range of motion. Flexibility exercises, like stretching and yoga, can help improve posture, prevent injuries, and enhance overall mobility.

## Flexibility Benefits

Flexibility offers numerous benefits, such as:

1. **Work-Life Balance**: Flexibility allows individuals to better balance their work and personal commitments, leading to reduced stress and improved overall well-being.

2. **Increased Productivity**: Allowing flexible work arrangements, like remote work or flexible hours, can boost productivity as employees can tailor their work schedule to their most productive times.

3. **Talent Attraction and Retention**: Offering flexibility can attract a wider pool of talent and help retain employees who value a better work-life balance.

4. **Cost Savings**: Flexible work arrangements can lead to reduced overhead costs for office space, utilities, and other resources.

5. **Global Workforce**: Flexibility enables organizations to tap into a global talent pool without the limitations of geographical boundaries.

6. **Diversity and Inclusion**: Flexibility supports employees with different needs, including parents, caregivers, and those with disabilities, fostering a more inclusive workplace.

7. **Employee Engagement**: Providing flexibility shows that employers value their employees' needs, leading to increased engagement and job satisfaction.

8. **Reduced Commuting Stress:** Remote work or flexible hours can alleviate the stress of commuting, resulting in better employee well-being.

9. **Health and Wellness**: Flexibility allows employees to better prioritize their health, leading to reduced burnout and improved mental health.

10. **Adaptability**: Flexible organizations can quickly adapt to changes in the business environment or unexpected disruptions.

11. **Reduced Turnover**: Employees are more likely to stay with a company that offers flexibility, reducing turnover costs.

12. **Environmental Impact**: Reduced commuting and office space usage can contribute to a smaller carbon footprint.

Overall, flexibility in the workplace fosters a healthier, happier, and more productive workforce, while also providing benefits for the organization's operations and bottom line.

## Aging's Impact on Flexibility

As we age, our muscles and connective tissues tend to lose elasticity and become stiffer. This is due to a combination of factors, including changes in collagen production, decreased physical activity, and the natural wear and tear our bodies experience over time. Additionally, joint fluid may decrease, affecting joint lubrication and flexibility. Regular physical activity, stretching, and maintaining a healthy lifestyle can help mitigate some of these effects.

## Elderly Flexibility Issues

As people age, several common flexibility issues can arise due to factors like decreased physical activity, muscle stiffness, and joint changes. Some of the most common flexibility issues for the elderly include:

**Reduced Joint Mobility:** Aging can lead to a decrease in joint lubrication and cartilage thinning, resulting in reduced joint range of motion. This can make movements less fluid and more difficult.

**Muscle Stiffness:** As muscles lose their elasticity with age, they become more prone to stiffness. This can hinder daily activities and increase the risk of injuries.

**Loss of Muscle Mass:** Age-related muscle loss, known as sarcopenia, can contribute to decreased muscle flexibility and strength. This can make it harder to perform tasks that require bending, reaching, or lifting.

**Balance Issues:** Reduced flexibility can impact balance, making seniors more susceptible to falls. Tight muscles can restrict the ability to make quick adjustments to maintain stability.

**Postural Changes:** Poor posture can lead to muscle imbalances and reduced flexibility. Over time, this can contribute to discomfort and difficulty moving freely.

**Joint Stiffness:** Aging joints may experience stiffness due to decreased synovial fluid production, leading to a feeling of "stuck" joints and limited movement.

**Tight Hamstrings:** The muscles at the back of the thighs can become tight with age, affecting the ability to bend at the hips and knees.

**Limited Spinal Flexibility:** Reduced flexibility in the spine can lead to discomfort and difficulty with activities that involve twisting or bending.

**Decreased Foot and Ankle Mobility:** Stiffness in the feet and ankles can affect walking and balance, increasing the risk of tripping and falling.

**Ligament and Tendon Changes:** Aging can lead to changes in the properties of ligaments and tendons, making them less pliable and flexible.

To address these flexibility issues, regular physical activity that includes stretching, range-of-motion exercises, and balance training is crucial. Consultation with a healthcare professional or a physical therapist can help create a tailored exercise plan that addresses the specific needs and limitations of the individual.

## Gender & Flexibility Difference

On average, men tend to have slightly less flexibility compared to women due to differences in muscle mass, joint structure, and hormonal influences. However, it's important to note that there is a wide range of flexibility within each gender, and individual variation can be significant. Flexibility can also be improved through regular stretching and exercise regardless of gender.

Here are some of the key gender differences in flexibility and their explanations:

1. **Muscle Mass and Distribution**: Men generally have higher muscle mass and greater muscle bulk due to higher levels of testosterone. This can limit their range of motion in certain joints and contribute to decreased overall flexibility.

2. **Joint Structure**: Women tend to have slightly different joint structures, such as wider hip joints, which can facilitate greater flexibility in areas like the hips and pelvis. Men, on the other hand, might have more stability in certain joints due to their different joint anatomy.

3. **Hormonal Influences**: Hormones, particularly estrogen, play a role in maintaining joint flexibility. Estrogen can increase the elasticity of connective tissues, which may contribute to women's increased flexibility. Men's lower estrogen levels might contribute to comparatively lower joint flexibility.

4. **Connective Tissue Composition**: Women often have more flexible and elastic connective tissues, such as ligaments and tendons, which can enhance their range of motion. Men's connective tissues are generally thicker and less elastic, potentially limiting their flexibility.

5. **Body Composition**: Women tend to have a higher proportion of body fat compared to men. This can provide additional cushioning around joints and allow for greater range of motion in some cases.

6. **Biomechanics and Movement Patterns**: Men and women might naturally adopt slightly different movement patterns due to their anatomical differences. These patterns can affect flexibility and joint mobility over time.

7. **Cultural and Social Factors**: Societal expectations and gender norms might influence how individuals of different genders approach

physical activities like stretching, yoga, or dance. Women might be more encouraged to engage in activities that promote flexibility.

It's important to note that these differences are general trends and that individual variations can be significant. Furthermore, flexibility can be improved through regular stretching exercises and training, regardless of gender.

## Stretching Types

Stretching are of different types, some of which are listed below:

1. **Static Stretching**: This involves holding a stretch for a prolonged period, usually around 15-60 seconds. It helps improve flexibility by lengthening muscles and increasing range of motion.

2. **Dynamic Stretching:** Dynamic stretches involve moving parts of your body through a full range of motion. It's often used as part of a warm-up routine to increase blood flow and prepare muscles for activity.

3. **Ballistic Stretching**: This type uses bouncing or jerking motions to push muscles beyond their usual range. It can be risky as it might lead to injury, so it's generally not recommended.

4. **Active Stretching**: This involves holding a position using the strength of the opposing muscles. It helps improve flexibility and strength simultaneously.

5. **Passive Stretching**: In passive stretching, an external force (like a partner, gravity, or an object) is used to push a joint or muscle into a stretched position. It can be effective but requires caution to avoid overstretching.

6. **PNF (Proprioceptive Neuromuscular Facilitation) Stretching**: PNF combines passive stretching and isometric contractions. It typically involves a partner and is often used in rehabilitation settings to improve flexibility and range of motion.

7. **Isometric Stretching:** This involves contracting a muscle without changing its length. It's often used to improve strength and flexibility at the same time.

8. **Yoga and Pilates**: These practices incorporate a combination of various stretching techniques, focusing on flexibility, balance, and strength.

Remember, it's important to choose the appropriate type of stretching based on your fitness level, goals, and any existing injuries. Always warm up before attempting any stretching routine, and listen to your body to avoid overstretching or causing injury.

## Testing Flexibility Methods

Flexibility testing is a way to assess a person's range of motion and the elasticity of their muscles and joints. It's often used in fitness, sports, and rehabilitation settings to measure and improve flexibility. Various tests and exercises can be employed to evaluate different muscle groups and joints.

Flexibility can be tested through various methods that assess the range of motion and suppleness of joints and muscles. Here are a few common tests and their explanations:

- **Sit-and-Reach Test**: This test measures the flexibility of the lower back and hamstrings. The individual sits on the floor with legs extended and tries to reach forward as far as possible. A measuring device determines how far they can reach.

- **Shoulder Flexibility Test**: In this test, the individual reaches one arm over their shoulder and the other arm behind their back, attempting to touch fingers. This assesses shoulder and upper body flexibility.

- **Trunk Rotation Test**: This test evaluates the flexibility of the spine. The person sits on the floor, knees bent, and twists their torso to one side while keeping hips square. The angle of rotation is measured.

- **Hip Flexor Test**: It measures the flexibility of the hip flexor muscles. The individual kneels on one knee while the other leg is extended forward. They then lunge forward to feel a stretch in the hip flexor region.

- **Ankle Flexibility Test**: This assesses the flexibility of the ankles. The individual sits with legs extended and ankles hanging off the edge of a bench. They flex their feet, attempting to point the toes upward.

- **Goniometer Measurements**: Goniometers are devices used to measure joint angles. By measuring the angles at which joints can move, such as the knee or elbow, flexibility can be assessed.

- **Yoga and Pilates Poses**: Various yoga and Pilates poses can be used as tests of flexibility. The ability to comfortably execute poses that require stretching and range of motion indicates flexibility.

- **Dynamic Stretching Routine**: Observing how well an individual performs a series of dynamic stretches, such as leg swings or arm circles, can provide insights into their flexibility.

- **Functional Movement Tests**: These involve assessing flexibility within functional movements, such as squatting or reaching overhead. The ease and range of motion during these movements can indicate overall flexibility.

- **Spinal Flexibility Test**: This test involves measuring the range of motion of the spine by observing how far an individual can bend forward, backward, and laterally.

Remember that flexibility is specific to different joints and muscle groups. A combination of these tests can provide a comprehensive understanding of an individual's flexibility and help identify areas that might require improvement. Always perform these tests under proper guidance and avoid overstretching to prevent injury.

## Stretching Recommendations

These are some general stretching recommendations:

1. **Warm Up**: Always start with a light warm-up before stretching to increase blood flow to the muscles.

2. **Dynamic Stretching:** Use dynamic stretches (controlled movements) before workouts to engage and activate muscles.

3. **Static Stretching**: Hold static stretches (stationary positions) after workouts when muscles are warm, aiming for 15-60 seconds per stretch.

4. **Breathing**: Breathe deeply and evenly while holding stretches to promote relaxation and flexibility.

5. **Focus on Major Muscle Groups**: Target major muscle groups like hamstrings, quadriceps, calves, hips, shoulders, and back.

6. **Gradual Progression**: Gradually increase the intensity and duration of your stretches over time.

7. **Pain-Free**: Stretch to the point of mild tension, never to the point of pain.

8. **Consistency**: Regular stretching is more effective than occasional intense sessions.

9. **Balance**: Stretch both sides of your body equally to prevent imbalances.

10. **Cool Down**: End with a cool-down period to allow your heart rate to gradually return to normal.

Remember that individual needs vary, so consulting a fitness professional or physical therapist can provide personalized guidance based on your goals and physical condition.

### 16 Great Static Stretches

Static stretches can help improve flexibility and mobility. Here are 16 great static stretches you can try:

1. Quadriceps Stretch: Stand near a wall or a piece of sturdy exercise equipment for support. Grasp your ankle and gently pull your heel up and back until you feel a stretch in the front of your thigh.

2. Hamstring Stretch: To stretch your hamstring muscles:
   - Lie on the floor near the outer corner of a wall or a door frame.
   - Raise your left leg and rest your left heel against the wall.
   - Gently straighten your left leg until you feel a stretch along the back of your left thigh.
   - Hold for about 30 seconds.
   - Switch legs and repeat.

3. Calf Stretch: While holding on to a chair, keep one leg back with your knee straight and your heel flat on the floor. Slowly bend your elbows and front knee and move your hips forward until you feel a stretch in your calf. Hold this position for 30 to 60 seconds.

4. Hip Flexor Stretch: Hip flexor stretch (edge of table)
   - Lie flat on your back on a table or flat bench, with your knees and lower legs hanging off the edge of the table.
   - Grab your good leg at the knee, and pull that knee back toward your chest. ...
   - Hold the stretch for at least 15 to 30 seconds.
   - Repeat 2 to 4 times.

5. Butterfly Stretch: To do the butterfly stretch:
   - Sit on the floor or a prop with the soles of your feet pressing into each other.
   - To deepen the intensity, move your feet closer in toward your hips.
   - Root down into your legs and sitting bones.
   - Elongate and straighten your spine, tucking your chin in toward your chest.

6. Glute Stretch: Sit on the floor and extend your legs in front of you. Keeping your back straight, lift your left leg and place your left ankle on your right knee. Lean slightly forward to deepen the stretch. Hold for 20 seconds, then repeat on the other side.

7. Triceps Stretch:
   - Bring your left elbow straight up while bending your arm.
   - Grab your left elbow with your right hand, and pull your left elbow toward your head with light pressure.
   - If you are more flexible, you may pull your arm slightly behind your head.
   - You will feel the stretch along the back of your arm.

8. Shoulder Stretch: While standing or sitting, and with your arms by your side and a straight back, slowly lift your shoulders up toward your ears. Hold here for a few seconds.

9.  Chest Stretch: To stretch the muscles of your chest:
    - Place your hands behind your head.
    - Squeeze your shoulder blades together, bringing your elbows back as far as possible.
    - Hold the stretch for 30 seconds.


10.      Upper Back Stretch:
    - Stretch your arms out in front of your body. Clasp one hand on top of your other hand.
    - Gently reach out so that you feel your shoulder blades stretching away from each other.
    - Gently bend your head forward.
    - Hold for 15 to 30 seconds.
    - Repeat 2 to 4 times.


11. Neck Stretch:
    - Turn your head gently to the right, and then gently to the left.
    - Remember not to strain your neck or push yourself to the point that you feel pain.
    - Hold the stretch for 2 to 3 seconds before moving your head to the opposite side.
    - Repeat this stretch 10 times in each direction, two times a day.


12. Seated Forward Bend:
    - Sit with your legs together or hip-width apart, and straight in front of you.
    - Make sure you are sitting high up on your sitting bones.
    - Inhale and reach with both arms toward the ceiling, arms parallel to your ears.
    - As you exhale, keep on reaching forward, and bend forward, reaching with your hands toward your toes.

13. Standing Forward Fold:
    1. Stand up tall and bend forward by rotating your hip joints.

2. Keep your knees straight and place your palms on the floor, or hold the back of your ankles.

3. Stay in standing forward bend pose for 30 seconds to 1 minute.

14. Child's Pose: Stretch your arms in front of you with the palms toward the floor or bring your arms back alongside your thighs with the palms facing upwards.

15. Lunge Stretch: At the bottom of the lunge, your knees should both be bent to approximately 90 degrees. Reach down with both hands so your fingertips are touching the floor

16. Standing Side Stretch:
    1. Stand up tall with your feet shoulder-width apart, hold a dumbbell with both hands, and raise your arms up and above your head.
    2. Bend your torso to the right, as far as it feels comfortable, and pause.
    3. Return to the initial position and bend to the left side.
    4. Keep alternating sides until the set is complete.

Remember to hold each stretch for about 15-30 seconds and breathe deeply while doing them. Make sure to warm up a bit before starting your stretching routine and consult a professional if you have any existing injuries or health concerns.

## Yoga For Flexibility

Yoga is a practice that focuses on both physical and mental well-being. When it comes to improving flexibility through yoga, there are specific poses and practices that can help. Here's a detailed explanation:

1. **Dynamic Warm-up:** Before attempting any poses, start with a gentle warm-up to increase blood flow to the muscles and prepare the body for movement. Gentle stretches and joint rotations can be effective.

2. **Standing Poses:** Poses like "Trikonasana" (Triangle Pose), "Utthita Parsvakonasana" (Extended Side Angle Pose), and "Virabhadrasana" (Warrior Poses) focus on opening the hips and stretching the sides of the body, thereby increasing flexibility.

3. **Forward Bends:** Poses such as "Uttanasana" (Standing Forward Fold) and "Paschimottanasana" (Seated Forward Bend) work on stretching the hamstrings, lower back, and spine.

4. **Backbends**: Backbending poses like "Bhujangasana" (Cobra Pose), "Ustrasana" (Camel Pose), and "Urdhva Mukha Svanasana" (Upward-Facing Dog Pose) help to open up the chest and shoulders, while also increasing flexibility in the spine.

5. **Twists**: Twisting poses like "Parivrtta Trikonasana" (Revolved Triangle Pose) and "Bharadvajasana" (Bharadvaja's Twist) enhance spinal mobility and flexibility in the torso.

6. **Hip Openers**: Poses like "Baddha Konasana" (Bound Angle Pose) and "Eka Pada Rajakapotasana" (Pigeon Pose) target the hip flexors, outer hips, and groin, promoting greater hip flexibility.

7. **Inversions**: Inverted poses such as "Adho Mukha Vrksasana" (Handstand) and "Sirsasana" (Headstand) challenge the body's balance and help improve flexibility in the shoulders and core.

8. **Props and Modifications**: Props like blocks, straps, and bolsters can be used to support the body in poses, making them accessible to individuals with varying levels of flexibility.

9. **Consistency**: Regular practice is key. Gradually increasing the duration and intensity of your practice will yield better results over time.

10.     **Mindful Breathing**: Focus on your breath while holding poses. Deep, controlled breaths can help relax tense muscles and aid in achieving a greater range of motion.

11. **Cool Down and Savasana**: Finish your practice with gentle stretches and a final relaxation pose called "Savasana." This allows the body to recover and integrates the benefits of the practice.

Remember that flexibility takes time to develop, and pushing yourself too hard can lead to injury. Listen to your body, avoid overstretching, and work within your comfort zone. If you're new to yoga or have any health concerns, consider consulting a yoga instructor or a healthcare professional before starting a new practice.

## Chapter 5
## **MOBILITY-MOVE IT OR LOOSE IT!**

Mobility is a key component of total fitness. It refers to the ability of your joints to move through their full range of motion without any discomfort or restriction. Incorporating mobility exercises into your fitness routine can improve flexibility, reduce the risk of injuries, and enhance overall functional movement. Examples of mobility exercises include dynamic stretches, yoga, foam rolling, and specific joint mobility drills. Remember to prioritize proper form and listen to your body while performing these exercises.

### **The Importance of Mobility**

Mobility is a crucial aspect of total fitness for several reasons:

1. Joint Health: Mobility exercises help maintain and improve the health of your joints. When you move your joints through their full range of motion, you promote the circulation of synovial fluid, which nourishes the joints and helps prevent stiffness and discomfort.

2. Injury Prevention: Improved mobility can reduce the risk of injuries by ensuring that your muscles, tendons, and ligaments are flexible and capable of handling various movements without strain or overexertion.

3. Functional Movement: Good mobility enables you to perform daily activities and functional movements more efficiently. It helps you bend, twist, lift, and carry objects with greater ease, enhancing your overall quality of life.

4. Posture and Alignment: Mobility exercises can correct imbalances in muscle length and strength, promoting better posture and alignment. This, in turn, reduces the likelihood of developing chronic pain or musculoskeletal issues.

5. Performance Enhancement: For athletes, improved mobility contributes to enhanced athletic performance. It allows for greater range of motion in sports-specific movements, leading to improved agility, speed, and power.

6. Recovery and Rehabilitation: Mobility exercises can aid in the recovery process after intense workouts or injuries. Gentle mobility work can increase blood flow to recovering muscles, helping to alleviate soreness and promote healing.

7. Flexibility and Muscle Activation: Mobility work often involves stretching, which helps improve flexibility. It also activates muscles that might be neglected during more traditional exercises, leading to a more balanced muscular development.

8. Mind-Body Connection: Mobility exercises encourage a mindful approach to movement. Paying attention to your body's sensations and limitations fosters a stronger mind-body connection, promoting self-awareness and self-care.

9. Aging Gracefully: Maintaining good mobility as you age can greatly impact your quality of life. It can help you retain your independence by allowing you to perform everyday tasks with ease.

10. Stress Relief: Engaging in mobility exercises can be relaxing and stress-relieving. Slow, controlled movements can help calm the nervous system and provide a mental break from the hustle and bustle of daily life.

Incorporating mobility exercises into your fitness routine can yield a wide range of benefits that complement other aspects of fitness, such as strength, endurance, and cardiovascular health. It's important to consult with a fitness professional or healthcare provider before starting a new exercise regimen, especially if you have any existing medical conditions or concerns.

# Typical Mobility Issues

Here are five typical mobility issues that can impact overall fitness:

1. **Joint Stiffness**: Stiff joints can limit your ability to move freely and perform exercises effectively, potentially leading to discomfort and reduced range of motion.

2. **Muscle Tightness**: Tight muscles can restrict movement and increase the risk of injuries during workouts, as well as impact your overall flexibility.

3. **Poor Posture**: Incorrect posture can affect your body alignment, leading to imbalances, reduced mobility, and an increased risk of pain or injuries.

4. **Limited Range of Motion**: Insufficient range of motion in joints can limit your ability to perform exercises correctly and prevent you from achieving full movement potential.

5. **Muscle Imbalances**: When certain muscle groups are stronger or tighter than others, it can lead to improper movement patterns, affecting mobility and increasing the risk of overuse injuries.

## Improving Your Mobility

Here are some ways to improve mobility as part of your total fitness routine:

1. Dynamic Stretching: Incorporate dynamic stretches before your workout to warm up and increase joint mobility.

2. Static Stretching: Perform static stretches after your workout to help maintain and improve flexibility.

3. Foam Rolling: Use a foam roller to release muscle tension and improve tissue mobility.

4. Yoga: Engage in regular yoga sessions to enhance flexibility, balance, and overall mobility.

5. Mobility Drills: Include mobility-specific exercises and drills that target problem areas.

6. Functional Movements: Focus on exercises that mimic real-life movements to improve overall mobility.

7. Joint Mobility Exercises: Perform exercises that specifically target joint mobility, such as hip circles and shoulder rotations.

8. Balance Training: Incorporate balance exercises to improve stability and coordination.

9. Regular Movement Breaks: Avoid prolonged periods of sitting; take short breaks to stand, stretch, and move around.

10. Pilates: Participate in Pilates classes to strengthen core muscles and improve flexibility.

11. Cross-Training: Engage in a variety of physical activities to challenge different muscle groups and movement patterns.

12. Proper Posture: Maintain good posture throughout the day to prevent stiffness and improve overall mobility.

13. Mobility Tools: Use tools like resistance bands and mobility balls to assist in improving range of motion.

14. Massage Therapy: Consider regular massages to help release muscle tension and improve circulation.

15. Hydration: Stay adequately hydrated to maintain joint lubrication and overall tissue health.

Remember, consistency is key when it comes to improving mobility. Gradually incorporate these practices into your routine and pay attention to your body's response. Always consult a fitness professional or healthcare provider before making significant changes to your exercise routine.

## Self-Myofascial Release

Self-myofascial release (SMR) is a technique that involves applying pressure to certain areas of the body using tools like foam rollers or massage balls to alleviate muscle tension, improve flexibility, and promote relaxation. It's often used as part of a warm-up or cooldown routine, and can be helpful for athletes, individuals with muscle tightness, or those seeking to enhance their overall mobility. Remember to use proper technique and listen to your body's feedback while performing SMR exercises.

## Dynamic Stretching

Dynamic stretching is a form of stretching that involves moving parts of your body through a full range of motion in a controlled and deliberate manner. It's commonly used as a warm-up activity in total fitness routines because it helps increase blood flow, improve flexibility, and prepare muscles for more intense exercises. Examples of dynamic stretches include leg swings, arm circles, and hip rotations. It's a valuable component of a well-rounded fitness routine.

Here are three examples of dynamic stretching exercises that can be incorporated into a total fitness routine:

- Leg Swings: Stand next to a wall or support, and gently swing one leg forward and backward in a controlled manner. This helps to improve flexibility in the hip and thigh muscles.

- Arm Circles: Extend your arms out to the sides and make circular motions with your arms. This can help to loosen up the shoulder joints and improve range of motion.

- Walking Lunges: Take a step forward into a lunge position, keeping your front knee directly above your ankle. Push off the front foot to return to a standing position and then repeat on the other leg. This exercise dynamically stretches the hip flexors and leg muscles.

Remember to perform dynamic stretches after a light warm-up to help prepare your muscles for more intense exercise.

### Mobility Drills For Fitness

These are a few mobility drills that can help improve your overall fitness:

1. Hip Circles: Stand with your feet hip-width apart and place your hands on your hips. Slowly make circles with your hips, moving them in a clockwise and then counterclockwise direction. This helps improve hip mobility.

2. Arm Swings: Stand with your feet shoulder-width apart and extend your arms out to the sides. Swing your arms in a circular motion, gradually increasing the size of the circles. This helps improve shoulder mobility.

3. Leg Swings: Find a stable support (like a wall or a pole) to hold onto. Swing one leg forward and backward while keeping the other leg straight. This helps improve hip and hamstring flexibility.

4. Ankle Circles: Sit on the floor with your legs extended. Lift one leg off the ground and make circular motions with your ankle. This improves ankle mobility and flexibility.

5. Cat-Cow Stretch: Start on your hands and knees in a tabletop position. Inhale as you arch your back (cow pose) and exhale as you round your back (cat pose). This helps improve spine flexibility.

6. Thoracic Rotation: Lie on your side with your knees bent and arms outstretched in front of you. Keeping your lower body stable, rotate your upper body to the opposite side. This helps improve rotational mobility in the upper back.

7. Deep Squat Hold: Squat down as low as you comfortably can with your feet flat on the ground and your elbows inside your knees. This helps improve hip and ankle mobility.

Remember to perform these mobility drills gently and gradually. They can be done as part of your warm-up routine or separately to improve your overall mobility and flexibility.

# Chapter 6
## STABILITY-FINDING THE BALANCE

Stability is an important aspect of total fitness. It refers to the ability of your body to maintain balance and control during various movements and activities. Incorporating exercises that focus on balance, core strength, and flexibility can help improve stability and overall fitness. This can include exercises like yoga, Pilates, balance training, and functional strength workouts. Remember to consult a fitness professional before making significant changes to your exercise routine.

## The Stability -Mobility Continuum Concepts

The Stability-Mobility Continuum is a concept in fitness that emphasizes the balance between stability and mobility within the body. It suggests that certain areas of the body need to be stable, while others require mobility. Achieving this balance helps prevent injuries and enhances overall fitness. For instance, the core and joints like the hips often need stability, while areas like the shoulders benefit from greater mobility. This concept guides exercise routines to address both stability and mobility for optimal fitness.

The Stability-Mobility Continuum in total fitness refers to a concept that classifies different exercises and movements based on their focus on stability or mobility. Here are the five points along this continuum:

1. Stability: Exercises that emphasize stability involve maintaining a steady base of support while performing movements. These exercises enhance core strength and balance.

2. Controlled Mobility: These exercises combine stability and controlled movement. They challenge your muscles to work together while maintaining control throughout the range of motion.

3. Dynamic Mobility: These movements involve greater ranges of motion and require joint flexibility and muscle activation. They aim to improve functional movement patterns.

4. Dynamic Stability: These exercises incorporate both stability and mobility elements. They focus on maintaining control while moving through various planes of motion.

5. Agility: Agility exercises emphasize rapid changes in direction, speed, and coordination. They improve reaction time, quickness, and overall athletic performance.

Remember that finding the right balance between stability and mobility is important for a well-rounded fitness routine.

## Keeping Our Body Stable

Maintaining body stability while staying fit involves focusing on core strength, balance exercises, and proper form during workouts. Incorporating activities like yoga, Pilates, and stability ball exercises can help enhance your stability and overall fitness. Remember to progress gradually to avoid injury and consult a fitness professional if you're unsure where to start.

Here are five ways to keep your body stable while staying fit:

1. Balanced Nutrition: Maintain a well-rounded diet that includes a variety of nutrients to support overall health and energy levels.

2. Regular Exercise: Engage in a consistent workout routine that combines cardiovascular activities, strength training, and flexibility exercises.

3. Hydration: Drink an adequate amount of water throughout the day to keep your body properly hydrated, especially during and after workouts.

4. Proper Rest: Ensure you get enough sleep to allow your body to recover and repair itself after physical activity.

5. Stretching and Warm-ups: Prioritize proper warm-ups and stretching to prevent injuries and improve flexibility, which contributes to stability.

Remember, everyone's body is different, so it's essential to listen to your own body's signals and adjust your approach accordingly.

## Improving Your Stability

Improving overall stability in your fitness routine involves a multifaceted approach:

1. **Core Strength**: Strengthen your core muscles through exercises like planks, Russian twists, and leg raises. A strong core stabilizes your body during various movements.

2. **Balance Training**: Incorporate balance exercises like single-leg stands, Bosu ball exercises, and stability ball movements. These challenge your proprioception and improve stability.

3. **Functional Movements**: Focus on functional exercises that mimic real-life movements. This enhances your body's ability to stabilize during everyday activities.

4. **Proper Form**: Maintain proper form during exercises. This prevents compensatory movements and reduces the risk of injury.

5. **Progressive Training**: Gradually increase the intensity and complexity of your workouts. This challenges your stability over time.

6. **Mind-Body Connection**: Develop a strong mind-body connection by paying attention to your body's movements and sensations during exercises.

7. **Yoga and Pilates**: These practices emphasize both strength and flexibility while enhancing stability and body awareness.

8. **Incorporate Unstable Surfaces:** Use balance boards, stability balls, or foam pads to introduce controlled instability into your workouts.

9. **Variation**: Include a variety of exercises that target different muscle groups and movement patterns.

10. **Recovery**: Allow time for proper recovery to prevent overuse injuries and maintain your body's ability to stabilize effectively.

Remember, consistency is key. Gradually integrating these strategies into your fitness routine will help improve your overall stability and enhance your fitness progress.

## Stability In Gym Routine

To add stability to your gym routine, consider incorporating exercises that focus on balance and core strength, such as planks, stability ball exercises, single-leg squats, and yoga poses. Additionally, using equipment like resistance bands, Bosu balls, and stability discs can challenge your stability and enhance your overall workout experience. Just remember to start with proper form and gradually increase intensity to avoid injury.

Here are five ways to maintain stability in your gym routine:

- Consistency: Stick to a regular workout schedule to build a routine that your body and mind can adapt to.

- Gradual Progression: Increase weights, intensity, or duration gradually to avoid overexertion and reduce the risk of injury.

- Balanced Workouts: Incorporate a variety of exercises that target different muscle groups to ensure overall strength and prevent imbalances.

- Proper Form: Focus on maintaining correct form during exercises to maximize effectiveness and minimize the risk of injuries.

- Rest and Recovery: Allow your body enough time to recover between workouts. Incorporate rest days and consider factors like sleep, hydration, and nutrition to aid in recovery.

# Chapter 7

## AGILITY-NOW THE FUN BEGINS

Agility refers to the ability to move quickly and easily, as well as the capacity to change direction rapidly and effectively. It's often associated with physical attributes, but the concept can extend to mental flexibility and adaptability too. In sports and business, agility is crucial for staying competitive and responding to changes in a dynamic environment.

### Agility Training Benefits

Agility training offers several benefits, including improved coordination, faster reaction times, enhanced balance, and increased flexibility. It's particularly useful for athletes and individuals looking to boost their performance in sports or daily activities that require quick movements and changes in direction. Regular agility training can also help prevent injuries by strengthening muscles and joints.

Here are 8 benefits of agility training:

1. Improved Coordination: Agility training helps enhance your ability to move quickly and smoothly, improving coordination between different parts of your body.

2. Enhanced Reaction Time: Regular agility exercises can lead to faster reaction times, crucial in various sports and everyday situations.

3. Increased Speed: Agility training can contribute to an overall increase in your speed and acceleration, beneficial for athletes and fitness enthusiasts.

4. Better Balance: Agility exercises challenge your balance, leading to improved stability and reducing the risk of falls and injuries.

5. Sports Performance: Agility training is particularly valuable for athletes, as it can directly improve their performance in sports that require quick changes in direction, such as soccer, basketball, and tennis.

6. Core Strength: Many agility exercises engage your core muscles, leading to a stronger core that supports overall body stability and posture.

7. Cardiovascular Fitness: Agility drills often involve bursts of high-intensity activity, which can contribute to improved cardiovascular fitness and endurance.

8. Mental Agility: The focus and concentration required during agility training can help enhance your cognitive skills and mental sharpness.

Keep in mind that individual results may vary, and it's important to tailor your training to your personal goals and physical abilities.

## Agility Training: Plyometrics

Agility training is a vital component of total fitness that aims to enhance an individual's ability to change direction quickly and efficiently while maintaining balance and control. It is particularly beneficial for athletes, as well as individuals seeking improved coordination and movement skills.

One method of agility training within total fitness is plyometrics. Plyometrics involves explosive, high-intensity movements that help improve power, speed, and coordination. It's a form of exercise that focuses on quick and forceful muscle contractions, often involving jumping, hopping, and bounding exercises.

Plyometric exercises typically consist of three phases:

1. **Eccentric Phase**: This is the pre-loading phase where muscles lengthen under tension. For example, in a squat jump, this is the phase where you lower your body into a squatting position before jumping.

2. **Amortization Phase**: This is the brief pause between the eccentric and concentric phases. It's the transition from muscle lengthening to muscle shortening. A shorter amortization phase is ideal for generating powerful movements.

3. **Concentric Phase**: This is the explosive contraction phase where muscles shorten, generating force and producing rapid movements. In a squat jump, this is the phase where you jump off the ground.

Plyometric exercises should be executed with caution to prevent injury. Proper technique and a gradual increase in intensity are essential. Here are some common plyometric exercises used in agility training:

1. **Box Jumps**: Jump onto and off of a box, focusing on using your legs and core to generate power and height.

2. **Depth Jumps**: Step off a platform, land softly, and immediately explode upward into a jump.

3. **Lateral Bounds**: Jump sideways from one foot to the other, emphasizing controlled movement.

4. **Skater Jumps**: Jump from side to side, mimicking the movement of a speed skater.

5. **Agility Ladder Drills**: Perform various footwork patterns in an agility ladder to improve quick foot movement and coordination.

6. **Bounding**: Perform exaggerated running steps, focusing on generating power and distance with each stride.

7. **Medicine Ball Throws**: Use explosive movements to throw a medicine ball against a wall or to a partner.

These exercises help develop the fast-twitch muscle fibers needed for rapid changes in direction and acceleration. When incorporating plyometrics into agility training, it's important to have a well-structured program that gradually increases intensity and includes proper warm-up and cool-down routines. Additionally, individual fitness levels and any existing injuries should be considered when designing a plyometric workout plan.

Chapter 8

# NUTRITION: YOU ARE WHAT YOU (CHOOSE) TO EAT

Nutrition is the process of obtaining and consuming essential nutrients from food to support growth, energy, and overall health. It involves macronutrients (carbohydrates, proteins, and fats) for energy and tissue building, as well as micronutrients (vitamins and minerals) for various bodily functions. A balanced diet that includes a variety of foods from all food groups is important for maintaining proper nutrition and preventing deficiencies or health issues.

## Nutrition and Aging

Nutrition plays a crucial role in the aging process. As we age, our metabolism changes, and nutrient needs can shift. A balanced diet rich in nutrients like vitamins, minerals, fiber, and protein can help maintain muscle mass, bone health, and cognitive function. Adequate hydration is also important. It's recommended to consult a healthcare professional or registered dietitian to create a personalized nutrition plan that addresses specific aging-related concerns.

## Nutrients Overview

Macronutrients are essential nutrients that your body needs in larger quantities. They include carbohydrates, proteins, and fats, providing energy and supporting various bodily functions. Micronutrients are required in smaller amounts and include vitamins and minerals, which play a crucial role in maintaining good health and proper bodily functions.

## Macro & Micronutrients

Here's a general list of macronutrients important for bodybuilders:

**Proteins**:

- Lean meats (chicken, turkey, beef)
- Fish and seafood
- Eggs
- Greek yogurt
- Cottage cheese
- Tofu and tempeh
- Whey protein powder

**Carbohydrates**:

- Whole grains (brown rice, quinoa, oats)
- Sweet potatoes
- Fruits (berries, apples, bananas)
- Vegetables (broccoli, spinach, kale)
- Legumes (beans, lentils, chickpeas)

**Fats**:

- Nuts and seeds (almonds, walnuts, chia seeds)
- Avocado
- Olive oil
- Fatty fish (salmon, mackerel)
- Nut butters (peanut butter, almond butter)

Remember, individual nutritional needs can vary, so it's a good idea to consult with a registered dietitian or nutritionist to create a personalized macronutrient plan that aligns with your specific goals and requirements.

## Micronutrients

Here are some essential micronutrients that are important for bodybuilders:

1. **Vitamin D:** Helps with muscle function and immune system support.

2. **Calcium**: Crucial for bone health and muscle contractions.

3. **Iron**: Necessary for oxygen transport and energy production.

4. **Magnesium**: Aids in muscle relaxation and protein synthesis.

5. **Zinc**: Supports immune function and protein metabolism.

6. **Vitamin C:** Helps with collagen formation and immune support.

7. **Vitamin E**: Acts as an antioxidant and supports muscle recovery.

8. **B Vitamins (B6, B12, Biotin, Folate)**: Assist in energy metabolism and nerve function.

9. **Omega-3 Fatty Acids**: Reduce inflammation and support heart health.

Remember, a balanced diet that includes a variety of nutrient-rich foods is crucial for optimal health and performance. It's always a good idea to consult a registered dietitian or nutritionist for personalized advice.

## Vegetables and Fruits To Keep Fit

Here are some vegetables and fruits that can be beneficial for keeping fit and Bodybuilding due to their nutritional content and potential health benefits:

**Vegetables:**

1. Spinach
2. Broccoli

3. Brussels sprouts
4. Kale
5. Sweet potatoes
6. Bell peppers
7. Cauliflower
8. Asparagus
9. Zucchini
10. Carrots

**Fruits:**

1. Berries (blueberries, strawberries, raspberries)
2. Bananas
3. Apples
4. Oranges
5. Pineapple
6. Mangoes
7. Kiwi
8. Watermelon
9. Pears
10. Grapefruit

Remember that a well-rounded diet is important for bodybuilders, including a mix of carbohydrates, proteins, healthy fats, and a variety of vitamins and minerals from different food sources. Always consult a registered dietitian or nutritionist for personalized advice based on your specific needs and goals.

## Whole Grains

Whole grains are an essential part of a balanced diet that contributes to overall fitness. Unlike refined grains, whole grains contain the entire grain kernel, including the bran, germ, and endosperm. This provides a greater amount of nutrients like fiber, vitamins, minerals, and antioxidants, which offer various health benefits such as improved digestion, better blood sugar control, and reduced risk of chronic diseases like heart disease and diabetes.

Here are some examples of whole grains:

1. Brown rice
2. Quinoa
3. Oats
4. Barley
5. Whole wheat (including whole wheat bread and pasta)
6. Buckwheat
7. Millet
8. Amaranth
9. Farro
10. Bulgur

Incorporating a variety of these whole grains into your diet can help enhance your overall fitness and well-being.

## Proteins

Proteins are essential macromolecules that play a crucial role in total fitness. They are composed of amino acids and are involved in various bodily functions, including muscle growth and repair, immune system function, enzyme activity, and hormone regulation. In the context of fitness, proteins are especially important for muscle development and recovery after workouts.

Examples of protein sources for total fitness include:

1. Lean meats like chicken, turkey, and beef.
2. Fish and seafood like salmon, tuna, and shrimp.
3. Eggs, which are a complete source of protein.
4. Dairy products such as Greek yogurt, cottage cheese, and milk.
5. Plant-based sources like beans, lentils, tofu, tempeh, and quinoa.

These protein-rich foods provide the amino acids necessary to support muscle growth, repair tissues, and maintain overall fitness levels. Remember that a well-balanced diet with a variety of protein sources is essential for optimal results in your fitness journey.

## Water

Water plays a crucial role in total fitness. Staying hydrated is essential for maintaining bodily functions, supporting energy levels, and aiding in recovery during and after exercise. Drinking water helps regulate body temperature, lubricate joints, and transport nutrients. It's important to drink water before, during, and after workouts to prevent dehydration and optimize performance. The exact amount of water needed varies based on factors like activity level, climate, and individual needs, but aiming for around 8 glasses (8 ounces each) a day is a common guideline.

The amount of water you need for Total Fitness per day can vary based on factors such as your age, gender, activity level, and climate. A common guideline is to aim for around 8 glasses of water per day (about 2 liters), but some individuals might need more. Listen to your body's signals and adjust your water intake accordingly to stay hydrated during your fitness routine.

## Electrolytes

Electrolytes play a crucial role in maintaining proper hydration and muscle function during physical activity. They include minerals like sodium, potassium, calcium, and magnesium. Consuming electrolyte-rich foods or drinks can help replenish these minerals lost through sweat and support overall fitness performance.

Electrolytes are minerals that carry an electric charge and are crucial for various bodily functions, especially during physical activity. Here are seven important electrolytes and their roles in total fitness:

- Sodium: Helps maintain fluid balance and supports nerve and muscle function. It's lost through sweat and needs to be replenished, especially during intense workouts.

- Potassium: Plays a role in muscle contractions, nerve function, and maintaining fluid balance. Adequate potassium levels can help prevent muscle cramps and support overall muscle health.

- Calcium: Essential for muscle contractions, including the heart, and helps maintain bone strength. It's important for overall muscle and skeletal health during exercise.

- Magnesium: Contributes to energy production, muscle contractions, and bone health. It can help reduce muscle soreness and cramps during and after workouts.

- Chloride: Works with sodium to maintain fluid balance and proper hydration. It's often found in salt and helps maintain the body's electrolyte equilibrium.

- Phosphate: Supports energy production and bone health. It's involved in ATP (energy molecule) production, important for sustaining physical activity.

- Bicarbonate: Helps regulate blood pH and maintain acid-base balance. During exercise, the body produces more carbon dioxide, which is buffered by bicarbonate to prevent overly acidic conditions.

Balancing these electrolytes is essential for optimal performance, preventing dehydration, and supporting overall fitness goals. Remember that individual electrolyte needs can vary based on factors such as exercise intensity, duration, and environmental conditions.

## Caloric Intake

Caloric intake is a crucial factor in overall fitness. To achieve your fitness goals, it's important to balance the calories you consume with the calories you burn through physical activity. If you're aiming to lose weight, you generally need to create a caloric deficit. If you're looking to gain muscle, you might need a caloric surplus. Consulting a nutritionist or fitness professional can help you determine the right caloric intake for your specific goals.

Here are 7 caloric intake concepts related to total fitness:

1. Maintenance Calories: This is the number of calories you need to consume to maintain your current weight. It's the balance point between the calories you burn through daily activities and the calories you consume through food.

2. Caloric Surplus: Consuming more calories than your maintenance level leads to a caloric surplus. This is often used for gaining muscle mass, as the extra calories provide the energy needed for muscle growth.

3. Caloric Deficit: Consuming fewer calories than your maintenance level results in a caloric deficit. This is commonly used for weight loss, as the body taps into its stored fat for energy, leading to gradual weight reduction.

4. Bulking: This involves intentionally entering a caloric surplus to promote muscle gain. It often includes weight training and proper nutrient intake to optimize muscle growth.

5. Cutting: Cutting refers to entering a caloric deficit to reduce body fat while maintaining muscle mass. This is usually combined with cardiovascular exercise and careful dietary planning.

6. Lean Gains: Lean gains focus on a small caloric surplus, aiming to slowly build muscle while minimizing fat gain. It's a balanced

approach that promotes muscle growth without excessive fat accumulation.

7. Refeeding: Refeeding involves temporarily increasing caloric intake, usually with carbohydrates, after a period of being in a caloric deficit. It helps to boost metabolism and provide psychological relief during weight loss efforts.

Remember, individual caloric needs vary based on factors like age, gender, activity level, and metabolism. Consulting with a registered dietitian or a fitness professional can help you determine the best caloric intake strategy for your fitness goals.

Sample Daily Menu

Here are a couple of sample daily menus that could fit within a total fitness plan. Remember, these are just examples and can be adjusted based on your dietary preferences, calorie needs, and fitness goals.

**Sample Daily Menu 1:**

**Breakfast:**

- Scrambled eggs with spinach and tomatoes
- Whole grain toast
- Greek yogurt with berries

**Lunch:**

- Grilled chicken salad with mixed greens, cucumbers, bell peppers, and a light vinaigrette dressing
- Quinoa or brown rice on the side

**Snack:**

- Apple slices with almond butter

**Dinner:**

- Baked salmon with lemon and herbs
- Steamed broccoli
- Sweet potato

## Sample Daily Menu 2:

**Breakfast:**

- Oatmeal topped with sliced bananas, chopped nuts, and a drizzle of honey
- Low-fat milk or plant-based milk alternative

**Lunch:**

- Turkey and avocado wrap with whole wheat tortilla
- Carrot and celery sticks with hummus

**Snack:**

- Mixed nuts and dried fruit

**Dinner:**

- Lean beef stir-fry with colorful vegetables (e.g., bell peppers, snap peas, carrots) in a light soy-ginger sauce
- Quinoa or whole grain noodles

Remember, these menus are just starting points. Focus on incorporating a balance of lean proteins, whole grains, healthy fats, and plenty of fruits and vegetables. Adjust portion sizes and food choices based on your specific needs and goals. It's also a good idea to consult with a registered dietitian or nutritionist for personalized guidance.

# Chapter 9
## WARM-UP, COOL DOWN & RECOVERY

### Warm-up and Cool down

Warm up and cooling down are important components of any workout routine. They help prepare your body for exercise and aid in recovery afterward. Here's a detailed explanation of both:

## Warming Up:

Warming up is the process of gradually preparing your body for more intense physical activity. The main goals of warming up are to increase your heart rate, improve blood circulation, enhance flexibility, and mentally prepare yourself for the workout ahead. Here's how to effectively warm up:

1. Cardiovascular Activity: Start with 5-10 minutes of low-intensity cardio, such as jogging, brisk walking, or cycling. This increases your heart rate and blood flow, gradually raising your body temperature.

2. Dynamic Stretching: Perform dynamic stretches that involve movement, like leg swings, arm circles, or hip rotations. This helps improve joint mobility and flexibility.

3. Sport-Specific Movements: Incorporate movements that mimic the activity you're about to perform. For instance, if you're doing a leg-focused workout, do some bodyweight squats.

## Cool Down:

Cool down is just as important as warming up. It's a way to gradually bring your body back to its normal state after a workout, reducing the risk of injury and aiding in recovery. Here's how to properly cool down:

1. Low-Intensity Activity: After your main workout, spend 5-10 minutes doing low-intensity cardio or gentle movements. This helps maintain blood flow to prevent blood pooling in your muscles.

2. Static Stretching: Incorporate static stretches, where you hold each stretch for about 15-30 seconds. Focus on the major muscle groups you targeted during your workout. This helps improve flexibility and reduce muscle tightness.

3. Breathing and Relaxation: Take a few deep breaths to help calm your body and bring your heart rate back to normal. This can also aid in reducing post-exercise tension.

**Why They're Important**:
Warming up gradually increases your heart rate, dilates blood vessels, and prepares your muscles for the upcoming workload. This can enhance performance, prevent injuries, and optimize energy utilization. Cooling down helps your body gradually transition from intense activity to a resting state. It aids in preventing muscle soreness, promoting circulation, and reducing the risk of dizziness or fainting after exercise.

Remember, the specific duration and intensity of warm-up and cool-down activities can vary based on factors such as your fitness level, the type of exercise, and your personal preferences. It's essential to tailor your warm-up and cool-down routine to suit your needs.

## Fitness Recovery Tips

"Fitness recovery" refers to the process of allowing your body to rest and repair after physical activity to optimize your overall fitness levels. It involves a combination of rest, nutrition, hydration, and other techniques to promote healing and growth. Here's a detailed breakdown of the key components:

1. Rest and Sleep: Adequate sleep is crucial for recovery. During deep sleep, the body releases growth hormone, which aids in muscle repair and tissue regeneration. Aim for 7-9 hours of quality sleep per night.

2. Nutrition: Proper nutrition is essential for recovery. After exercise, your body needs protein to repair and build muscles, and carbohydrates to replenish glycogen stores. Hydration is also vital to replace fluids lost during sweating.

3. Hydration: Staying hydrated helps maintain optimal bodily functions and supports recovery. Water aids in nutrient transport, temperature regulation, and waste removal.

4. Active Recovery: Light exercises like walking, yoga, or swimming at a low intensity can enhance blood flow to muscles, reducing muscle soreness and promoting recovery.

5. Stretching and Mobility Work: Gentle stretching and mobility exercises can improve flexibility and reduce the risk of injury. They also help increase blood flow to muscles, assisting in the removal of waste products.

6. Foam Rolling and Massage: Foam rolling can help release muscle tension and knots, improving circulation and reducing muscle soreness. Professional massages also aid in muscle recovery.

7. Cold and Heat Therapy: Alternating between ice baths and warm baths/showers can improve circulation, reduce inflammation, and alleviate muscle soreness.

8. Mind-Body Techniques: Techniques like meditation and deep breathing can reduce stress levels, which can impact recovery. Lower stress levels contribute to better sleep and overall well-being.

9. Periodization: Varying the intensity and volume of your workouts over time can prevent overtraining and reduce the risk of injuries. Incorporate rest days and lighter training periods into your routine.

10.      Listen to Your Body: Pay attention to how your body feels. If you're consistently fatigued, experiencing persistent muscle soreness, or lacking motivation, it may be a sign that you need more recovery.

11. Professional Guidance: If you're engaged in intense training or have specific fitness goals, consulting a fitness professional or a coach can help tailor a recovery plan to your individual needs.

Remember that recovery is an integral part of any fitness journey. It allows your body to adapt to the stresses of exercise, preventing burnout and injuries, and ultimately improving your overall fitness and performance.